The Principle Approach Diet Handbook

How to Stop Counting Calories, Carbs, and Points to Follow Six Practical Principles to Develop Your Own Program for Ideal Weight and Improved Health

By Debra Wechter
Illustrated by HollySueStudio

Dedication

This handbook is dedicated to everyone who knows that they are a slim person imprisoned in an overweight body and truly believes that they will break free from that prison when they only find a way.

Author's Testimony

These principles are the result of struggling myself with overweight as a teenager and young adult. I tried multiple diet programs but found them to be too restrictive to follow. However, on that journey I finally gained wisdom about what really works for the long haul and was able to lose thirty pounds and keep it off, even through three pregnancies, for the past 40+ years!

After witnessing the struggles of the overweight at a weight-loss support group that I attended with a family member, I decided to put the wisdom I have gained into a book that hopefully will help countless others to experience the success that I have experienced. I would like to encourage the reader to begin to put these principles into practice and enjoy the journey to the new you!

"Whether therefore ye eat, or drink, or whatsoever ye do, do all to the glory of God."

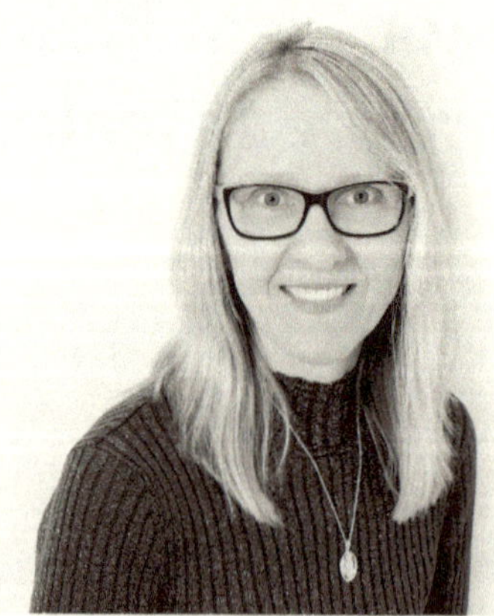

I Corinthians 10:31

Other People's Programs

Weight Watchers, Atkins, Medifast, Nutrisystem . . . the list of weight-loss programs is endless. Many of us have tried several of them, only to regain the weight when we return to our regular eating habits. Why is this so? It is because it is someone else's program we are following and not our own. A better way is to develop our own diet program using principles based upon sound nutrition and common sense that will work for a lifetime.

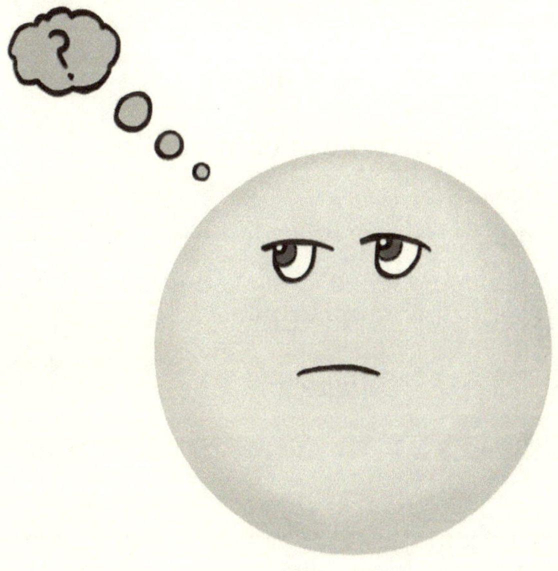

The Six Practical Principles of the Program

Principle #1

Ditch the Diet Mentality

Going on a weight-loss diet precedes going off a weight-loss diet, causing your weight to rise and fall with no permanent success. Instead adhere to principle number two . . .

Principle #2

Embrace a Permanent Lifestyle Change

Begin your permanent lifestyle change by asking yourself how you should eat for the rest of your life based upon sound nutrition and common sense that will result in obtaining your ideal weight and improved health. Then practice that change permanently!

Principle #3

Focus on Food - Not Weight

Have you ever cleared a cobweb from a corner of your living room, only to have it reappear the following day? You forgot to get rid of the spider! With the spider still present the web returns. So it is with our weight. We may shed some pounds, but if we do not get rid of the "spider" of our bad eating habits, the weight quickly returns. Focus on what and when to eat and developing proper eating habits, and you will be delighted when you do step on the scale, which should not be more than once a week.

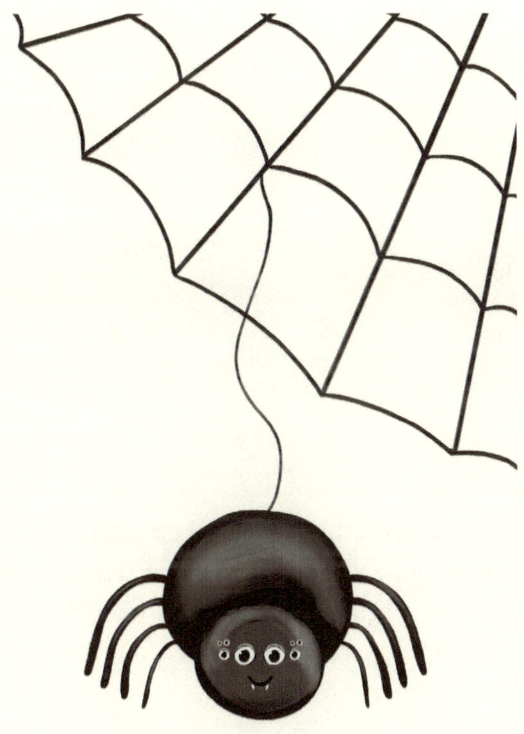

Principle #4

Establish an Eating Pattern

Eating at regular intervals each day will keep you feeling full and satisfied as well as help to establish and maintain a healthy metabolism. It will also help you to gain control of your eating habits and keep it. Because constant eating is a major cause of overweight, the eating pattern is very important. The suggested pattern is as follows:

BREAKFAST

SNACK

LUNCH

SNACK

DINNER

Allow two to three hours between each one. For example, you may eat breakfast at 7:00 am, snack at 10:00 am, lunch at 12:30 pm, snack at 3:00 pm, and dinner at 6:00 pm. You're done!

Principle #5

Stop Eating Early Evening

It has been said that what you eat after dinner you wear the next day. There is undoubtedly a lot of truth to that! Our bodies need fuel during the day when we are the most active but less at night as we prepare to sleep. It is best to discontinue eating early in the evening, then resume eating again the next morning after a minimum of a twelve-hour fast.

Weight loss may also occur more rapidly if the biggest meal of the day is eaten at midday instead of in the evening.

This schedule may need to be adjusted if you work nights or have some other circumstances that would make this schedule difficult to follow. The important thing is that you are eating at regular intervals throughout a twelve-hour period.

Principle #6

Follow a Low-Fat, High-Fiber Diet

You are probably asking yourself by now what you are supposed to eat on your own program. What do you like the most? Be sure to include it!

Foods that are low in fat and high in fiber make the best choices. Low-fat foods tend to be healthier and lower in calories. High fiber foods are also healthier, make us feel fuller, and help keep our digestive system functioning properly. Following a starch-based diet and eating a variety of foods from plants is the best way to accomplish this principle.

Two books that are very helpful in how to follow a starch-based diet are The McDougall Program - Twelve Days to Dynamic Health by John A. McDougall, M.D. (Copyright 1990) and The Rice Diet Solution by Kitty Gurkin Rosati, M.S., R.D., L.D.N., and Robert Rosati, M.D. (Copyright 2006).

If you love sweets and desserts like me, choose from the vast variety of low-calorie choices that are now available in your local supermarket in the snack food aisle or the frozen food section. Ice cream lovers should choose low-fat yogurt or reduced fat ice cream. Just be sure to measure the serving size with a measuring cup or your favorite mug.

A copy of the recommended food pyramid is also included in the back of this handbook.

Other Practical Pointers

It is common knowledge that there needs to be a calorie deficit in order to lose weight. Plan your meals carefully, avoiding second helpings and measuring serving sizes as needed.

You can eat anything you want but not everything you want (at the same time)! Balance is a key factor.

Practice mindful eating! Slow down, eliminate distractions, and pay close attention to what you are eating. It takes about twenty minutes for your mind to register that you are full.

Drinking water can also help you lose weight! It's calorie free, helps you burn more calories, and water may even suppress your appetite if consumed before meals.

Always be sure as well to read the label on packaged foods before buying or eating them. Check the fat grams and main ingredients. Many packaged foods need to stay on the store shelf or end up in the trash!

Another factor to consider for weight loss and maintenance is adequate sleep. When you are overtired, you tend to eat more and have less control. Try to get at least seven or eight hours of sleep every night.

These principles refer to your normal, daily diet whether you are eating at home, at work, or out in public. Holidays, birthdays, and other special occasions are times to relax and enjoy the foods that accompany the event. Just get back on your program the next day after the occasion!

Please Don't Say Exercise

Many of us cringe at the word exercise. We feel guilty about our lack of it and frustrated about how to make it a regular part of our busy lives. At least try to incorporate exercise into your daily life by doing things like taking walks, taking the stairs instead of the elevator, and even pacing when you are on the phone instead of sitting. Choosing something that you know you love like dancing or being involved in a sport can also make incorporating exercise into our lives less difficult. Whatever you choose remember this - keep moving!

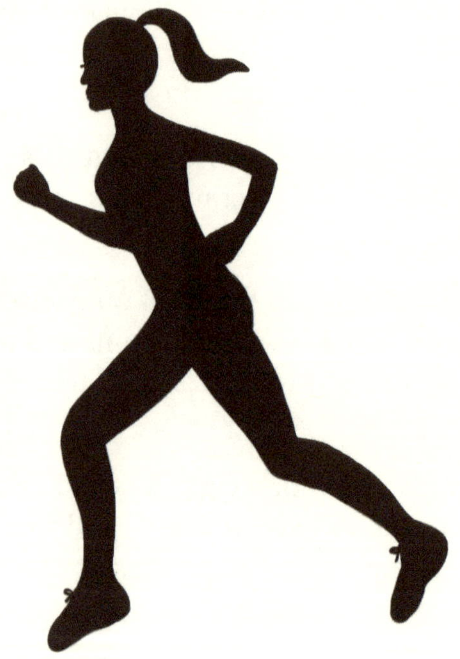

Suggested Food Choices

Protein

Meat, Fish,Poultry, Eggs, Nuts, Beans

Choose low-fat choices that are baked, broiled, boiled, microwaved, or grilled. Crock pot cooking is also acceptable with light marinades. Avoid frying whenever possible. If you do fry anything, use zero-calorie cooking spray. Beans of all kinds make an excellent low-fat alternative to meat choices even as a main dish. Protein shakes, which have become very popular, make a great healthy choice for a meal as well!

Grains

Whole grain breads and cereals that are high in fiber and nutrients make the best choices. Hot cereals such as oatmeal and cream of wheat cannot be beat for giving you a healthy, low-fat, high-fiber start to your day. Try adding raisins, fruit, or nuts to them for added fiber and nutrients.

Pasta that is either whole grain or enriched makes a good base for a healthy meal. Serve it with marinara sauce and low-fat meat or vegetables mixed in. Top with low-fat or grated parmesan cheese if desired. Pasta also makes a great salad choice when mixed with a variety of raw vegetables, seasoned lightly with salt and pepper or a table blend, and marinated with lite Italian dressing.

Regarding rice, brown rice is a much healthier choice than white rice because the fiber and nutrients are retained. Mix it with low-fat meat and/or vegetables for a nutrient packed meal.

Vegetables and Fruits

Oh, the luxury of vegetables and fruits! Any fresh or frozen vegetables and fruits can be added to your diet almost limitless as long as there are no added sugars or fats.

Fresh vegetables such as cauliflower, broccoli, carrots, etc., are great to eat raw with a low-fat dip. Canned vegetables are acceptable as long as the sodium content is not too high and there is no added sugar. Canned fruits are acceptable as well as long as they are canned in their own juices. Frozen vegetables and fruits are often better than canned when they do not contain added ingredients. Just be sure to check the label to see if there are any added ingredients or preservatives.

Even potatoes are actually low in fat and high in fiber and make a great dietary choice as long as they are not smothered in butter or covered with gravy. Try spraying them with zero-calorie spray butter or topping them with low-fat sour cream and season with a salt-free table blend instead.

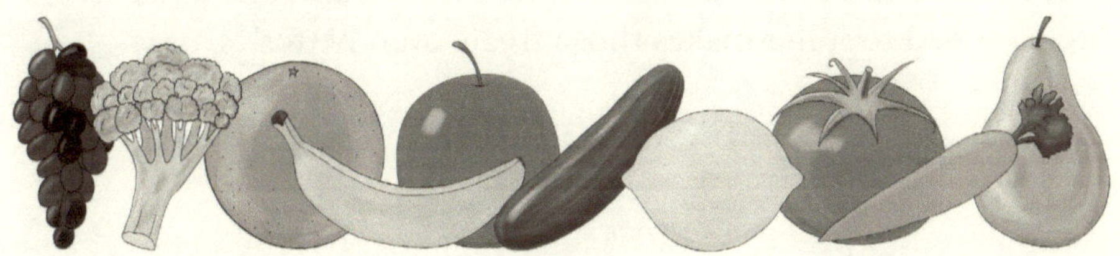

Dairy

Drink or cook with skim, low-fat, almond, or soy milk. Use cheese of any kind sparingly or choose low-fat options when available. Low-fat yogurt or reduced fat ice cream make great desserts if eaten in small amounts. Frozen treats on a stick provide a controlled amount and can satisfy a sweet tooth. A small amount of fat-free or lite whipped topping makes those treats even better!

Fats

A little fat goes a long way, so whatever you are using, use sparingly!

 Zero-calorie and zero-fat cooking sprays have fortunately replaced the need to fry with butter, oil, or grease. Reduced-fat margarines and zero-calorie spray butters make great substitutes for high-fat butter choices. Lite or reduced-fat mayonnaise or lite dressings make a great choice for sandwiches or salads over the high-fat options.

The list for proteins, grains, vegetables and fruits, dairy, and fats could go on and on. Just remember to think low fat, high fiber when making food choices!

Beverages

Be careful not to sabotage your efforts to lose weight with high calorie, sugary drinks with no nutritional value. Water with lemon or drink mixes sweetened with Stevia are two examples of better beverage choices. Carbonated waters with natural flavors make great choices as well. Beware, however, of drinks that have been sweetened with unhealthy artificial sweeteners such as aspartame. Check the label before purchasing any low-calorie drinks!

A beverage tip is to fill your glass with ice before adding any beverage, especially if it is not a zero-calorie beverage. When your drink is empty, then refill it with water only. A hint of the flavor of the previous beverage will still be present without adding any additional calories!

Enjoy the Journey

Have you attempted to follow many different weight-loss programs? You are not alone. Glean what you can from having done so and incorporate what you learned from them into your own program. Make the choice to develop your own program around the six principles, and enjoy the journey to the very best you! Here are the six principles again:

1. DITCH THE DIET MENTALITY

2. EMBRACE A PERMANENT LIFESTYLE CHANGE

3. FOCUS ON FOOD NOT WEIGHT

4. ESTABLISH AN EATING PATTERN

5. STOP EATING EARLY EVENING

6. FOLLOW A LOW-FAT, HIGH-FIBER DIET

Epilogue

Eating Pattern Sample Menus

Women follow as shown.

Men may increase portion sizes.

Low calorie hot beverages may be included with any meal.

Breakfast

1 Protein

1 Grain

1 Fruit

1 Dairy

Breakfast Examples

1 egg

1 piece of wholegrain toast with spray butter

4 ounces tomato juice

1 cup low-fat milk

OR

Protein Shake

made with:

1 cup low-fat milk

3 ice cubes

1 cup frozen fruit

1 scoop protein powder

Mix all ingredients in blender until smooth.

OR

1 cup cereal - hot or cold

1/2 cup or 1 fruit

1 cup low-fat milk

Lunch

1 Protein

2 Grains

2 Vegetables/Fruits

1 Dairy

1 Low-Calorie Drink

Lunch Examples

Sandwich made with:

2 ounces low-fat lunch meat

2 slices of wholegrain bread or 1 roll

tomato slices

chopped onions

1 slice cheese

2 teaspoons low-fat mayonnaise

1 ounce veggie chips

ice water with lemon

1/2 cup or 1 fruit

OR

Chicken Noodle Soup made with:

8-10 cups chicken broth

12 ounces egg noodles

1 cup chopped carrots

1 cup chopped celery

1/2 cup chopped onions

2 cups cooked chicken

Combine all ingredients and boil on low until everything is tender.

Recommended serving size - two cups. Sprinkle lightly with mozzarella cheese if desired.

Dinner

4 - 6 Ounces Protein

1 Grain

2 Vegetables/Fruits

1 Low-Calorie Drink

1 Low-Calorie Dessert

Dinner Examples

4 - 6 ounces skinless, boneless chicken breast

1 baked potato with spray butter

1/2 cup mixed vegetables

1 garden salad with lite Italian dressing

8 ounce drink sweetened with stevia

1/2 cup low-fat ice cream

Chicken made with:

Lite Italian Dressing

Place 3 - 5 pounds of skinless, boneless chicken breasts in crockpot. Cover with 8 - 16 ounces of lite Italian dressing. Cook for several hours until tender. Raw vegetables may be added during the cooking process.

OR

Ground Turkey/Tomato Soup made with:

1 pound ground turkey

6 cups beef broth

1 can 28 ounce diced tomatoes with basil, garlic, and oregano

1/4 cup chopped onions

1 can 15 ounce kidney beans, drained and rinsed, OR

6 ounces egg noodles or macaroni noodles

Fry ground turkey until fully cooked and crumbled. Add all remaining ingredients and boil on low until everything is tender.

Recommended serving size - two cups. Sprinkle lightly with parmesan cheese if desired.

Sample Snacks

1 fresh fruit

1 cup canned or frozen fruit

1 pouch fruit snacks

1 cup raw vegetables

1 low calorie granola bar

1 cup dry cereal

1 small yogurt

1 cheese stick

1 ounce veggie chips

1 ounce pop chips

1 ounce pretzels

1 ounce baked potato chips

1/2 cup mixed nuts

2 cups popcorn

2 rice cakes

Reflection Section

Principle # 1

Ditch the Diet Mentality

What diets have you tried, and what could you glean from them to help you develop your own program? Write down below what you would like to incorporate from them into your own diet program.

____

____

____

____

____

____

____

____

____

____

____

____

Principle # 2

Embrace a Permanent Lifestyle Change

How ready are you to embrace a permanent lifestyle change? Remember that today is the first day of the rest of your life! Write down your feelings below and solidify your commitment to yourself to make healthy eating lifestyle changes permanent!

Principle # 3

Focus on Food - Not Weight

It's so easy to focus on weight instead of foods that we are actually eating that cause us to be overweight. Write down below your current weight and goal weight, then set it aside until your eating pattern is fully established with better food choices. Make it a habit of only weighing yourself once a week or once every other week.

____

____

____

____

____

____

____

____

____

____

____

____

____

Principle # 4

Establish an Eating Pattern

Are you being successful in establishing an eating pattern and sticking to it? Indiscriminate eating, which is eating randomly without being able to remember what or when you ate, surely leads to weight gain! If evenings are a problem, try saving your light dessert for a little later beyond dinner. Perfection is not the goal, but the eating pattern and overnight fast is crucial! Write down below your current eating pattern with times noted, and keep track of your pattern for several days.

____

____

____

____

____

____

____

____

____

____

____

____

Principle # 5

Stop Eating Early Evening

How late in the evening are you still eating? Remember to stop eating early evening! A good goal is to be finished with dinner no later than 8:00 pm. Write down below the times that you finished eating entirely for the day for the next several days.

Principle # 6

Follow a Low-Fat, High-Fiber Diet

What have become your favorite low-fat, high-fiber food choices? Write those down below, and be sure to make them a regular part of your grocery list when you do your weekly shopping. Be on the lookout for new and exciting choices and update your list regularly.

As always, remember to follow the star and enjoy the journey!

____

____

____

____

____

____

____

____

____

____

____

____

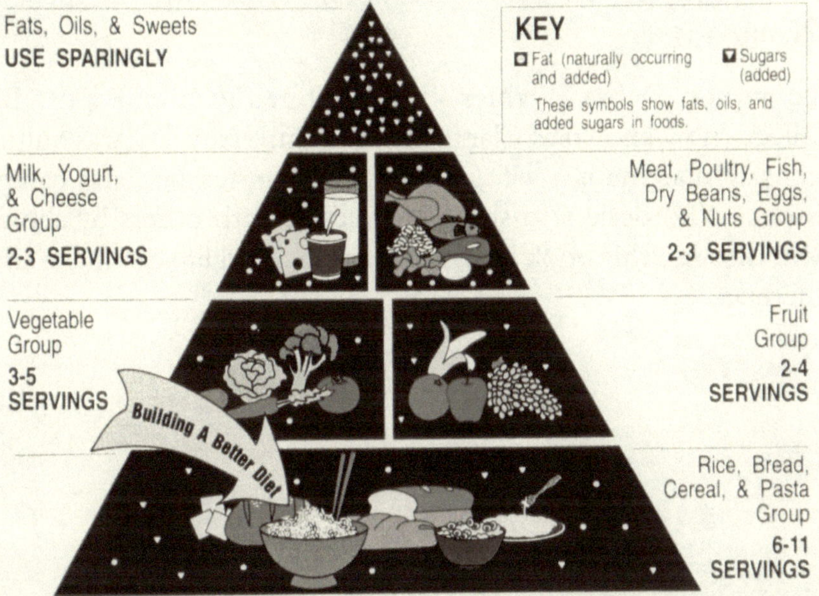

The Pyramid is a daily guide to help you choose from a variety of foods and in a proportion to help you build a better diet.

Weight loss diets abound, but they rarely produce the lasting results that the person is seeking. In this book the author proposes a new approach to weight loss and maintenance by modifying our eating habits permanently while following six practical principles daily. These principles can lead to the lasting results that the person is seeking.

The author, Debra Wechter, is a 1980 graduate of Baptist Bible College (now known as Clarks Summit University), Clarks Summit, Pennsylvania. She is a wife, mother of three, teacher, and paraprofessional who desires to share her success with others by showing them through this book how living a principled life can make all the difference.

www.ingramcontent.com/pod-product-compliance
Lightning Source LLC
Chambersburg PA
CBHW051239250726

48656CB00003B/1028